FUNCTIONAL MEDICINE PRINCIPLES

A Complete Guide For Navigating The Depths Of Wellness Through Insights And Unlocking The Secrets To Optimal Health

WALTER ZYAIRE

DISCLAIMER

The information in this book is intended only for general informational purposes; it should not be used in lieu of professional advice or medical care. Since the author is not licensed to practice therapy, the information offered should not be used in place of the expertise, judgment, or guidance of qualified mental health or medical professionals. Readers are encouraged to consult therapists, medical specialists, or other qualified authorities regarding their particular situation and needs. The publisher and author disclaim all liability for any actions or decisions taken by readers based on the information in this book. Results may vary from person to person and this book's approaches, procedures, and strategies may not be suitable in all circumstances. Considering unique situations and consulting a qualified expert are essential when choosing the right course of action. Neither the publisher nor the author recommend or guarantee the efficacy of any therapy or treatment that is indicated in this book. Because the information is based on the author's research and understanding at the time of publishing, it could not reflect the most recent developments or practices in the treatment area. The publisher and the author both disclaim all liability for the accuracy, completeness, or use of the material in this book. Readers bear full responsibility for the decisions and actions they choose in light of the information presented in this book.

TABLE OF CONTENTS

ABOUT THE BOOK

The Functional Medicine Principles book is a highly influential work in the field of wellness and healthcare. There is a growing recognition of the limitations of traditional approaches in managing complicated health concerns as the medical landscape continues to change. This book is a great resource for scholars, healthcare professionals, and anybody looking for a more comprehensive understanding of health and well-being because of its thorough examination of functional medicine principles.

To help readers understand functional medicine's significance in the larger framework of healthcare, the book's introduction clearly defines the field and lays out its goals. Through an exploration of the Foundations of Functional Medicine's philosophical underpinnings and historical evolution, the book offers practitioners a strong foundation for understanding the fundamental ideas that inform their approach to patient treatment.

The book focus on systems biology approach highlights how different body systems are interrelated and advances a comprehensive knowledge of health. The next chapter's examination of genetics and epigenetic emphasizes the value of personalized medicine by providing details on how health therapies are unique to each patient.

The practical application of the principles of functional medicine is enhanced by the chapters on balancing hormones, gut health, and nutritional medicine. Through discussing the effects of diet on health, the significance of gut health, and methods for hormone balance, the book provides medical professionals with practical knowledge that they may use in their daily work.

Furthermore, the book's dedication to a thorough and patient-centered methodology is seen in the inclusion of chapters on Mind-Body Medicine, Environmental Medicine, and Detoxification and a Patient-Centered Approach.

Real-world examples are given on Case Studies and Practical Applications, which shows how functional medicine ideas can be successfully applied to common health conditions.

 This book is an invaluable resource for anyone looking to learn more about the fundamentals of functional medicine. Its significance goes beyond conventional medical procedures, providing a paradigm change in favor of a more individualized and integrative approach to healthcare. This book is a valuable tool for healthcare professionals navigating the complexity of modern medicine because of its thorough examination of fundamental ideas and real-world applications.

CHAPTER ONE

OVERVIEW OF FUNCTIONAL MEDICINE PRINCIPLES

AN EXPLANATION AND SYNOPSIS OF FUNCTIONAL MEDICINE

A patient-centered, holistic approach to healthcare, functional medicine focuses on finding and treating the underlying causes of illnesses and imbalances in the body. Functional medicine aims to identify the underlying causes of a patient's health problems, as opposed to traditional medicine, which frequently uses medication to address symptoms. The aforementioned approach acknowledges the interdependence of the body's systems and underscores the significance of tailored and preemptive healthcare.

Fundamentally, functional medicine sees the body not as a collection of discrete symptoms but as a dynamic, complex system with interrelated pieces. To obtain a thorough understanding of a patient's health, practitioners of Functional Medicine take into account the patient's genetics, environment, lifestyle, and distinct biochemistry. This comprehensive study targets the particular variables causing a person's health difficulties, enabling a more focused and successful treatment strategy.

Promoting optimal performance and correcting internal imbalances are at the heart of functional medicine. These values include realizing that the body can repair itself with the correct assistance, appreciating the significance of a nutritious and well-balanced diet, and appreciating the influence of lifestyle elements like stress, sleep, and physical activity on general health.

A strong patient-practitioner relationship is essential to functional medicine since it allows patients to take an active role in their treatment and be empowered to make decisions about their health.

PRINCIPLES OF FUNCTIONAL MEDICINE ARE IMPORTANT

Functional medicine places a strong emphasis on preventive care. Functional medicine seeks to maximize health and well-being proactively by detecting and treating possible health concerns before they show symptoms. This proactive strategy frequently entails dietary adjustments, lifestyle adjustments, and individualized treatment regimens catered to the patient's specific requirements. By using this method, Functional Medicine aims to support resilience and long-term health in addition to symptom relief.

The potential for functional medicine concepts to offer a more complete and efficient healthcare model is what makes them so important. Functional medicine offers a more individualized and long-lasting approach to well-being by comprehending the interconnection of multiple body systems and addressing the underlying causes of health concerns. By encouraging a greater awareness of one's own body and a sense of personal responsibility for one's health, the patient-centered paradigm enables people to actively participate in their health.

Functional medicine is a paradigm change in healthcare that emphasizes fostering optimal function, identifying the underlying causes of health problems, and adopting a patient-centered approach. Its focus on preventative and individualized care is in line with promoting long-term health and well-being in addition to symptom management. Functional medicine is a promising way to address the complexity of human health and give people the tools to maximize their resilience and vitality as the field develops.

CHAPTER TWO

THE BASICS OF FUNCTIONAL MEDICINE

EVOLUTION IN HISTORY

A paradigm change in healthcare that departs from the conventional disease-centered concept is represented by functional medicine. Its roots in integrative and holistic medicine can be found in the 20th century when it began to evolve historically. The foundations of Functional Medicine were shaped in large part by pioneers like Dr. Jeffrey Bland, who emphasized the significance of treating the underlying causes of illness rather than only treating its symptoms.

This method was developed in response to the shortcomings of traditional medicine, which frequently concentrates on treating symptoms without addressing the underlying causes of illness.

IMPORTANT IDEAS AND CONCEPTS

The fundamental ideas and concepts that set functional medicine apart from the traditional medical paradigm are what drive it. Understanding that every person is unique and has a unique biochemical makeup impacted by genetic, environmental, and behavioral factors is one of the fundamental principles. A one-size-fits-all strategy might not be successful, therefore practitioners can customize interventions to meet the unique needs of each patient with the help of this individualized approach.

The interdependence of the body's systems is another of the tenets of functional medicine. Functions and organs are not seen in isolation; rather, Functional Medicine takes into account the complex web of connections among different physiological processes. With the use of this systems biology approach, practitioners may recognize and treat imbalances that could present as a variety of symptoms affecting several organ systems.

A fundamental tool for organizing and comprehending the complexity of a person's health is the Functional Medicine Matrix. This matrix includes all of the major clinical imbalances, including lifestyle decisions, environmental factors, genetic predispositions, and physiological processes. Through the process of charting these variables on the matrix, professionals can methodically examine how various components interact and pinpoint trends that may be responsible for a patient's health issues.

In the Functional Medicine Matrix, assimilation, defense and repair, energy, biotransformation and elimination, transport, communication, and structural integrity are the seven fundamental physiological activities that constitute the basis for comprehending health and illness. This framework makes it easier to investigate a patient's health in depth, which enables professionals to spot dysfunctional regions and create focused interventions to bring the patient's status back into balance.

A paradigm change in healthcare has been made possible by the historical development of functional medicine, which is founded on holistic methods and was pioneered by visionary individuals. Root cause analysis, systems biology, and customized treatment are the main tenets and philosophies. As a thorough tool, the Functional Medicine Matrix offers an organized framework for examining and addressing the complexity of health by taking into account the interdependent network of variables affecting a person's overall health.

CHAPTER THREE

A SYSTEMS BIOLOGY PERSPECTIVE

RECOGNIZING THE WHOLE HUMAN BODY

The systems biology approach, which emphasizes a comprehensive understanding of biological systems rather than separate components, marks a paradigm change in the study of the human body. This approach acknowledges that the human body is an intricately linked web of biological systems and processes that work in concert to preserve homeostasis. Researchers and medical professionals can better understand physiological processes, disease mechanisms, and therapeutic approaches by having a holistic view of the body and the dynamic interplay between its many components.

RELATIONSHIPS AMONG BODY SYSTEMS

The focus of systems biology is on recognizing the complex interdependencies among bodily systems.

This method takes into account the dynamic interactions and feedback loops that exist between various physiological systems rather than seeing organs and tissues in isolation. For example, to control blood pressure and oxygen levels, the cardiovascular system works closely with the respiratory and endocrine systems.

Determining the underlying causes of diseases, which frequently show up as disturbances in numerous systems, requires an understanding of these interdependencies. Researchers can find novel biomarkers and therapeutic targets by dissecting these intricate networks, opening the door to more individualized and successful treatment plans.

SYSTEMS THEORY IN FUNCTIONAL MEDICINE

Functional medicine's incorporation of systems thinking is an example of a modern approach to healthcare that goes beyond traditional reductionist paradigms. Functional medicine looks at the complex interplay of genetic, environmental, and lifestyle factors that affect health to treat diseases at their core. This approach is informed by the concepts of systems biology. Functional medicine attempts to bring back the balance and functionality of the complete biological system, as opposed to just treating symptoms.

This method places a strong emphasis on individualized and patient-centered care while accounting for each person's particular genetic composition and environmental exposures. Functional medicine offers a more proactive and all-encompassing approach to healthcare by adopting a systems thinking perspective. This approach focuses on optimizing general well-being and preventing diseases rather than merely treating individual illnesses.

By highlighting holistic viewpoints, acknowledging the interdependence of body systems, and encouraging systems thinking in functional medicine, the systems biology approach revolutionizes our understanding of the human body.

This paradigm change fosters a more integrated and personalized approach to understanding, preventing, and treating complex diseases, which has significant consequences for biomedical research and healthcare.

CHAPTER FOUR

GENETICS AND EPIGENETICS' ROLE

GENETIC AFFECTS ON HEALTH

There has been much investigation and study conducted on the influence of genetics on an individual's health. The basic building blocks of heredity, genes, are essential for defining a person's vulnerability to specific diseases and how they react to external stimuli, among other elements of their health. Genetic changes that are inherited may increase one's susceptibility to illnesses including diabetes, heart disease, and some types of cancer. The relationship between genetics and health is intricate, with many genes interacting to affect a person's general health.

Genetic research has advanced to the point where particular genes linked to different health disorders have been identified. Genetic testing has developed into a useful tool for determining a person's risk for developing specific diseases and for taking preventative action to lower that risk. But it's crucial to understand that non-genetic variables, lifestyle decisions, and the environment all have a big impact on how people's health turns out. Genetics is just one piece of the picture. Our awareness of the role that genetics plays in health is being further expanded by the developing discipline of genomic medicine, which opens the door to more individualized and focused approaches to treatment.

CHANGES IN EPIGENETICS

Changes in gene activity that do not result in modifications to the underlying DNA sequence are referred to as epigenetic changes. These alterations have the power to activate or deactivate genes and are essential for several biological functions. Histone alterations, non-coding RNA molecules, and DNA methylation are examples of epigenetic modifications. An individual's health and development are shaped by a dynamic layer of regulation that is influenced by lifestyle choices, experiences, and environmental circumstances.

The influence of early life events and environmental exposures on long-term health outcomes has been emphasized by research in the field of epigenetic. Throughout a person's life, epigenetic changes can take place, and comprehending these mechanisms has significant ramifications for both illness prevention and treatment. Further, as treatments that target particular epigenetic pathways may provide new ways to treat diseases with underlying epigenetic components, epigenetic research has revealed possible therapeutic paths.

IN FUNCTIONAL MEDICINE, PERSONALISED MEDICINE

A paradigm change in healthcare is represented by personalized medicine, especially when it comes to functional medicine. It moves away from a one-size-fits-all strategy and towards a more customized and focused form of care. To develop individualized treatment strategies, functional medicine takes into account each patient's distinct genetic and biochemical composition in addition to their lifestyle and surrounding circumstances. This method acknowledges the significance of treating the underlying causes of illness and adjusting interventions to meet the unique requirements of every person.

 Genetic data is important when it comes to personalized medicine. Through genetic testing, medical professionals can find genetic differences that could affect a person's reaction to a certain drug, their susceptibility to a particular ailment, and their overall risks to health. A more thorough understanding of a patient's health profile is made possible by integrating genetic insights with functional medicine concepts, which results in more efficient and individualized treatment plans.

CHAPTER FIVE

DIETARY MEDICINE

NUTRITION'S EFFECT ON HEALTH

An individual's total health and well-being are greatly influenced by their diet. Nutrition has a substantial effect on health, affecting many physiological systems and playing a major role in the development or prevention of a wide range of health disorders. The vital components needed for the body to function at its best are provided by a diet that is well-balanced and rich in nutrients. These components include vitamins, minerals, proteins, lipids, and carbs. Sufficient food intake boosts immunity, increases vitality, and preserves healthy organ function.

Beyond only providing for survival, diet also has a significant impact on the prevention of chronic illnesses including diabetes, heart disease, and some forms of cancer. A diet rich in whole grains, fruits, vegetables, and lean meats has been linked to a lower incidence of several disorders. On the other hand, unhealthy eating habits, which are defined as consuming large amounts of processed foods, sweets, and harmful fats, are linked to the development and advancement of several health problems.

NUTRITIONAL METHODS IN FUNCTIONAL MEDICINE

A holistic approach to healthcare is embraced by functional medicine, which emphasizes treating the underlying causes of health problems while acknowledging the interdependence of many body systems. Dietary strategies in the field of functional medicine emphasize individualized nutrition programs made to meet each person's specific requirements.

To create successful nutritional therapies, functional medicine practitioners take into account variables including heredity, lifestyle, and environmental impacts rather than using a one-size-fits-all strategy.

Finding and removing possible dietary sensitivity or intolerances that may be causing inflammation or other health problems is a common task in functional medicine. Furthermore, the focus is placed on optimizing the body's natural healing capabilities by supporting a varied and nutrient-dense diet. The incorporation of nutritional treatment into functional medicine highlights the significance of food as medicine and acknowledges its capacity to alter gene expression, impact metabolic pathways, and enhance general well-being.

SUPPLEMENTATION AND DEFICIENCY OF NUTRIENTS

Inadequate food intake, poor absorption, or elevated demand brought on by specific medical disorders can all result in nutrient deficiencies. Insufficiencies in vital vitamins and minerals can cause a variety of health issues, ranging from immune system dysfunction and exhaustion to more serious ailments like anemia or neurological abnormalities.

A crucial component of nutritional medicine is identifying and treating vitamin deficits.

When food sources aren't able to supply enough of a particular nutrient, supplements become essential. But it's crucial to use caution while supplementing, taking into account each person's needs as well as any possible drug interactions. Without the right supervision, taking too many supplements can cause imbalances and negative side effects.

There is no denying that diet has a profound effect on health, affecting both the molecular and systemic levels of the organism. Dietary approaches in functional medicine place a strong emphasis on tailored interventions; yet, correcting nutrient deficiencies through supplementation necessitates a sophisticated understanding of individual needs and associated hazards. Promoting optimal health and preventing a wide range of chronic diseases can be greatly aided by using a mindful and holistic approach to nutrition.

CHAPTER SIX

GUT CONDITION AND MICROBIOTA

THE VALUE OF GUT HEALTH

Because gut health has a direct impact on many physiological systems in the body, it is essential for preserving overall well-being. The gut microbiome, which is made up of bacteria, viruses, fungi, and other microorganisms, is a complex ecology that lives in the gastrointestinal (GI) tract. For the best possible immune system, nutrition absorption, and digestion, these microorganisms must be balanced and diverse. Intestinal problems including irritable bowel syndrome (IBS) and inflammatory bowel diseases (IBD) can be avoided in part by maintaining a healthy gut.

Furthermore, the body's energy balance is impacted by the gut as it is the main location for nutrition metabolism and synthesis. The synthesis of several vitamins, including vitamin K and B vitamins, which are necessary for several physiological processes, is also influenced by the gut microbiota. Numerous health problems, including obesity, diabetes, and autoimmune illnesses, have been connected to imbalances in the gut microbiota. Thus, preserving gut health is essential for both digestive health and general systemic health.

THE FUNCTION OF THE MICROBIOME IN HEALTH

The varied population of microorganisms that live in and on the human body is referred to as the microbiome, with the gut microbiome being one of the most intricate and significant.

The gut microbiome, which consists of billions of microorganisms, plays a major role in immunological and metabolic processes. The breakdown of dietary fibers and the fermentation of undigested carbohydrates are aided by beneficial bacteria in the gut, which results in the production of short-chain fatty acids (SCFAs), which support gut health and have anti-inflammatory properties.

Additionally, the microbiome serves as a barrier against the colonization of pathogenic organisms by generating antimicrobial chemicals and engaging in resource competition. It also has a major part in teaching the immune system how to discriminate between friends and enemies.

Dysbiosis, a term used to describe disruptions in the microbiome's equilibrium, has been linked to several illnesses, such as gastrointestinal problems, autoimmune diseases, and allergies.

Changes in the microbial composition of the gut microbiome have been related to mood disorders and neurological illnesses, highlighting the importance of this microbiome in impacting mental health. Because the gut and other body systems are interconnected, it is critical to preserve a varied and balanced microbiome for general health and well-being.

GUT-BRAIN RELATIONSHIP

The two-way communication between the central nervous system and the gastrointestinal tract is represented by the gut-brain connection. Neural, hormonal, and immunological networks facilitate this complex communication, which affects both physical and mental health. Often called the "second brain," the enteric nervous system is a sophisticated network of neurons buried in the gut wall that may function both independently and in constant communication with the central nervous system.

Because it produces metabolites and neurotransmitters that can affect brain function, the gut microbiome is essential to the gut-brain relationship. For instance, the gut flora affects the synthesis of serotonin, a neurotransmitter linked to mood control. The relationship between mental health conditions like anxiety and depression and imbalances in the gut microbiome highlights the significance of gut health for emotional well-being.

On the other hand, gut function can be impacted by stress and emotional emotions, which can result in modifications to intestinal permeability and microbial composition. The significance of addressing both gastrointestinal and mental health for overall well-being is highlighted by this bidirectional connection, which emphasizes the holistic character of health. Understanding and fostering the gut-brain link are becoming essential elements of a holistic approach to treatment, as research in this area progresses.

CHAPTER SEVEN

NATURAL HORMONE BALANCING

OVERVIEW OF THE ENDOCRINE SYSTEM

The endocrine system, a sophisticated network of glands that create and release hormones, is essential to the regulation of many physiological processes that occur within the body. Via the bloodstream, these chemical messengers affect organ and tissue function while preserving general homeostasis. The thyroid, pituitary, adrenal, and reproductive glands are important endocrine system actors that cooperate to maintain the delicate hormone balance required for optimum health.

HEALTH PROBLEMS AND HORMONE IMBALANCES

When particular hormones are present in excess or insufficient amounts, it can lead to hormone imbalances, which upset the delicate balance needed for healthy body operation. These imbalances can show up as several health problems, impacting mood, metabolism, the health of the reproductive system, and more. Fatigue, weight gain or loss, mood fluctuations, irregular menstruation cycles, and disturbed sleep habits are typical signs of hormone abnormalities.

PRACTICAL METHODS FOR HORMONE BALANCE

Naturally correcting hormone imbalances requires implementing practical strategies that prioritise enhancing general health. Hormone production and regulation depend on certain nutrients, which mean that nutrition plays a critical role in maintaining hormonal balance. A diet high in complete foods, such as vegetables, fruits, lean meats, and healthy fats, gives the body the building blocks it needs to synthesize hormones.

Another essential component of hormone balancing naturally is regular exercise.

Exercise contributes to overall hormonal balance by lowering stress, promoting the release of endorphins, and regulating insulin levels. Since the body's circadian rhythm affects the secretion of hormones like melatonin and growth hormone, which are essential for restorative activities during sleep, getting enough sleep is equally important.

Stress control is essential for maintaining hormone balance because long-term stress can cause the overproduction of cortisol, which can interfere with the endocrine system's normal ability to function. Deep breathing exercises, yoga, and meditation are examples of mind-body techniques that can reduce stress and support a more hormonally balanced environment.

Hormone balance is also influenced by environmental influences. Hormone synthesis and regulation can be disrupted by exposure to endocrine-disrupting chemicals, which are present in several plastics, insecticides, and personal care products. A healthier endocrine system can be achieved by limiting exposure to environmental toxins, opting for natural and organic goods, and using them.

 Including adaptogenic herbs in one's regimen is a comprehensive strategy for achieving natural hormone balance. Adaptogens, which include holy basil, rhodiola, and ashwagandha, have been demonstrated to support general endocrine function and assist the body's ability to adjust to stimuli. You can drink these herbs as supplements or make tinctures and drinks with them.

Restoring hormone balance by natural means necessitates a comprehensive strategy that takes into account many facets of the environment and lifestyle. A person's endocrine system can be strengthened by emphasizing sleep, exercise, stress reduction, nutrition, and reducing exposure to environmental contaminants. This will improve overall health and reduce the likelihood of hormone-related disorders.

CHAPTER EIGHT

DETOXING AND ENVIRONMENTAL HEALTH

THE BODY'S DETOXIFICATION PATHWAYS

The human body has complex detoxification systems in place that are essential for getting rid of dangerous substances and preserving general health. The gastrointestinal tract, skin, kidneys, liver, and lungs are the main organs involved in these routes. Particularly important to detoxification is the liver, which goes through several chemical steps to process and neutralize pollutants.

Toxins that are soluble in fat are transformed into intermediate molecules in Phase I, which are then conjugated to become soluble in water in Phase II for simpler clearance. Whereas the gastrointestinal system eliminates toxins through bowel movements, the kidneys filter and eliminate waste materials that are soluble in water.

Furthermore, by eliminating specific toxins through perspiration and breathing, the skin and lungs aid in detoxification.

HEALTH AND ENVIRONMENTAL TOXINS

Exposure to environmental pollutants has become an everyday occurrence in modern culture, leading to several health issues. These toxins can come from artificial chemicals found in food, household goods, and personal care products, as well as pollutants found in the air, water, and soil. Long-term exposure to environmental pollutants has been connected to several health concerns, such as elevated risk of chronic diseases, neurological disorders, respiratory problems, and endocrine disruption. Some compounds that can build up in the body over time and endanger general health are industrial chemicals, pesticides, heavy metals, and persistent organic pollutants. The effects of these poisons on health highlight the significance of efficient detoxification techniques in contemporary medicine.

DETOXIFICATION TECHNIQUES IN FUNCTIONAL MEDICINE

A holistic approach to health is taken by functional medicine, which emphasizes the interdependence of all body systems and addresses the underlying causes of health problems, including toxicity. In functional medicine, detoxification techniques include dietary changes, targeted supplements, and lifestyle adjustments. A change in diet may entail consuming nutrient-dense foods like cruciferous vegetables, berries, and herbs like turmeric that boost liver function. Frequent activity encourages perspiration, which helps the skin remove toxins. Maintaining kidney function and aiding in the elimination of waste materials that are soluble in water require enough hydration.

Furthermore, certain supplements like antioxidants and glutathione precursors could be suggested to improve the body's capacity to neutralize and get rid of pollutants. Effective stress-reduction strategies, like as mindfulness and getting enough sleep, are essential for promoting the overall detoxification processes. Individualized approaches are prioritized in Functional Medicine, taking into account the distinct genetic, environmental, and lifestyle factors that impact an individual's ability to detoxify.

CHAPTER NINE

MENTAL-PHYSICAL MEDICINE

RELATIONSHIP BETWEEN PHYSICAL AND MENTAL WELLBEING

A key component of mind-body medicine is the relationship between mental and physical health, highlighting the complex interactions between psychological and physiological well-being. Several studies have demonstrated the reciprocal relationship, showing how physical and mental healths are strongly correlated and how one can greatly influence the other. Chronic stress, worry, or depression, for example, can cause physical symptoms that aggravate problems including immune system malfunction, gastrointestinal disorders, and cardiovascular diseases.

On the other hand, physical illnesses can lead to or worsen mental health problems, which emphasize the significance of treating health as a holistic process.

TECHNIQUES FOR REDUCING STRESS

In mind-body medicine, stress reduction techniques are essential because they provide a comprehensive approach to addressing the interdependence of mental and physical health. These methods include gradual muscle relaxation, biofeedback, deep breathing exercises, and mindfulness meditation, among many other activities. In particular, mindfulness has drawn a lot of attention due to its potent ability to reduce stress. People can develop a more adaptive reaction to stressors by encouraging present-moment mindfulness and acceptance, which can have a good impact on both mental and physical health outcomes.

COMPLEMENTING FUNCTIONAL MEDICINE WITH MIND-BODY METHODS

Recognizing the interdependent relationship between the mind and body, the integration of mind-body therapies into functional medicine signifies a paradigm change in the field of medicine.

According to functional medicine, symptoms are signs of underlying systemic imbalances in the body rather than being distinct entities. By addressing both physical symptoms and the psychological and emotional factors that contribute to general health, mind-body practices can be included in this approach.

To achieve maximum health and well-being, this integration places a strong emphasis on individualized and patient-centered care, taking into account each person's particular experiences, lifestyle, and stressors.

Mind-body techniques are seen in functional medicine as complementary instruments that support the body's inherent healing capacities. Depending on the individual needs of each patient, these practices may involve lifestyle adjustments, treatments, and self-care techniques.

Functional medicine seeks to enable people to take an active role in their treatment by promoting collaborative interaction between medical professionals and patients.

This approach emphasizes a thorough grasp of the interconnection between the mind and body while acknowledging the significance of mental and emotional variables in determining physical health outcomes.

CHAPTER TEN

PATIENT-CENTERED METHODOLOGY

STRENGTHENING THE BOND BETWEEN PHYSICIAN AND PATIENT

Several core ideas that place a high priority on the patient's health and active involvement in their treatment are what define the patient-centered approach in healthcare. The development of a solid doctor-patient connection is one important factor. For patients and healthcare providers to collaborate, trust, and communicate effectively, this relationship is essential. Developing a good relationship with patients creates a space in which they feel comfortable disclosing vital health information, leading to more precise diagnoses and individualized treatment regimens.

A key component of developing a solid doctor-patient relationship is effective communication. Building trust through honest and open communication enables patients to voice their worries, pose inquiries, and take an active role in health-related conversations. Actively hearing patients' viewpoints and including them in the decision-making process fosters a cooperative relationship in healthcare.

TAILORED TREATMENT STRATEGIES

A key element of the patient-centered approach is customized treatment programs. Understanding that every patient is different, medical professionals work to develop individualized treatment plans that take the patient's medical background, preferences, and lifestyle into account. This method stresses the necessity for individualized therapies to address particular health challenges while acknowledging the uniqueness of patients. Healthcare practitioners can increase the probability of patient adherence and favorable health outcomes by personalizing treatment regimens.

The Patient-Centered Approach's customized treatment regimens incorporate a comprehensive understanding of patients in addition to medical measures. This entails taking into account their socioeconomic status, cultural beliefs, and individual preferences. Healthcare practitioners can improve patient outcomes by customizing treatment plans to fit each patient's unique circumstances and increase the effectiveness and relevance of therapies.

PATIENTS' EMPOWERMENT IN THEIR HEALTH JOURNEY

A crucial component of the patient-centered approach is empowering patients to take charge of their healthcare. Giving patients the knowledge, tools, and encouragement they need to actively participate in health-related decisions is a key component of empowerment. By participating in collaborative decision-making, healthcare providers make sure patients are aware of their illnesses and available treatments. Patients who feel empowered are more likely to accept responsibility for their health, follow treatment recommendations, and alter their lifestyles in ways that improve their general well-being.

Promoting health literacy and giving patients information are both essential components of patient empowerment. For people to understand medical information and make educated decisions regarding their care, healthcare providers are essential. Patients can be empowered to actively manage their diseases, take part in preventive measures, and alter their lifestyles in ways that improve their long-term health through education and support programs.

The Patient-Centered Approach places a high emphasis on the value of customized treatment regimens, patient empowerment, and strong doctor-patient relationships. Together, these ideas support a paradigm for healthcare that actively engages people in their health journeys, honors the individuality of every patient, and encourages collaboration.

CHAPTER ELEVEN

CASE STUDIES AND REAL-WORLD IMPLEMENTATIONS

SUCCESS STORIES IN FUNCTIONAL MEDICINE IN REAL LIFE

Functional medicine has proven effective in treating a wide range of health disorders with individualized treatment programs because of its holistic and patient-centered approach. An important illustration is the treatment of long-term conditions like diabetes. Functional medicine looks at the underlying causes of illness rather than just treating its symptoms, taking into account things like genetic predispositions, lifestyle choices, and nutrition. This technique is beneficial as evidenced by the better outcomes and long-term well-being that patients frequently experience.

A further noteworthy case study focuses on the effective use of functional medicine in treating autoimmune illnesses. While the main goal of traditional medication may be to suppress symptoms, functional medicine places more emphasis on locating and reducing the triggers that lead to autoimmune reactions. Patients have reported reduced frequency and severity of flare-ups along with symptom improvement by targeted supplementation, stress management, and dietary adjustments.

USING THE PRINCIPLES OF FUNCTIONAL MEDICINE TO ADDRESS COMMON HEALTH ISSUES

The concepts of functional medicine can be successfully used to treat common health problems that arise in routine clinical practice. Digestive health is one of these areas. The complex interactions that exist between nutrition, gut microbiota, and general health are taken into account in functional medicine. For example, those with irritable bowel syndrome (IBS) could benefit from a multimodal strategy that incorporates stress management, probiotics, and dietary changes. By restoring gut equilibrium, this customized approach seeks to alleviate symptoms beyond those of traditional symptomatic therapies.

Another area where the ideas of functional medicine can be very helpful is mental health. Functional medicine investigates the complex relationships between dietary inadequacies, lifestyle variables, and the gut-brain axis, instead of focusing only on psychiatric medicines. Combining techniques like cognitive-behavioral therapies with nutritional psychiatry has shown potential in the treatment of mental health issues including depression and anxiety, encouraging a more all-encompassing and long-term route to mental health.

OBSTACLES AND SOLUTIONS IN THE PRACTICE OF FUNCTIONAL MEDICINE

Despite the growing popularity of functional medicine, practitioners encounter some obstacles when attempting to incorporate this approach into traditional healthcare.

The time-consuming aspect of functional medicine consultations is one major obstacle. Compared to standard consultations, completing thorough assessments, going over long patient histories, and creating customized treatment plans take more time. To solve this, some practitioners use cutting-edge scheduling techniques, collect data using technology, and collaborate across disciplines to optimize workflows without sacrificing patient care.

The conventional medical community's low acceptance and comprehension of functional medicine presents another difficulty. It will need teamwork, efficient communication, and educational initiatives to close this gap. Functional and conventional medicine can work together more readily if functional medicine ideas are incorporated into medical curricula, communication between various healthcare paradigms is encouraged, and successful case examples are presented.

Functional medicine's effectiveness in treating chronic illnesses is demonstrated by successful real-world cases, and its adaptability to common health problems is demonstrated by its use. Notwithstanding obstacles, persistent endeavors to optimize procedures and augment cooperation portend opportunities for the sustained expansion and assimilation of functional medicine into conventional medical methodologies.